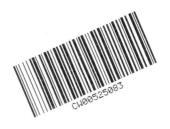

My Keto Air Fryer Recipes Collection

Super Simple Recipes

to Help You Lose Weight

Lydia Gorman

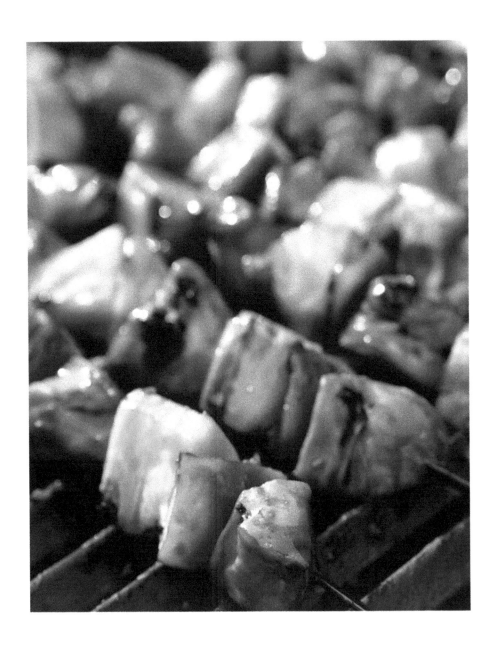

The following Book is reproduced below with the goal of providing information that is as accurate and reliable as possible. Regardless, purchasing this Book can be seen as consent to the fact that both the publisher and the author of this book are in no way experts on the topics discussed within and that any recommendations or suggestions that are made herein are for entertainment purposes only. Professionals should be consulted as needed prior to undertaking any of the action endorsed herein.

This declaration is deemed fair and valid by both the American Bar Association and the Committee of Publishers Association and is legally binding throughout the United States.

Furthermore, the transmission, duplication, or reproduction of any of the following work including specific information will be considered an illegal act irrespective of

if it is done electronically or in print. This extends to creating a secondary or tertiary copy of the work or a recorded copy and is only allowed with the express written consent from the Publisher. All additional right reserved.

The information in the following pages is broadly considered a truthful and accurate account of facts and as such, any inattention, use, or misuse of the information in question by the

Table of Contents

Introduction

What's the difference between an air fryer and deep fryer? Air fryers bake food at a high temperature with a high-powered fan, while deep fryers cook food in a vat of oil that has been heated up to a specific temperature. Both cook food quickly, but an air fryer requires practically zero preheat time while a deep fryer can take upwards of 10 minutes. Air fryers also require little to no oil and deep fryers require a lot that absorb into the food. Food comes out crispy and juicy in both appliances, but don't taste the same, usually because deep fried foods are coated in batter that cook differently in an air fryer vs a deep fryer. Battered foods needs to be sprayed with oil before cooking in an air fryer to help them color and get crispy, while the hot oil soaks into the batter in a deep fryer. Flour-based batters and wet batters don't cook well in an air fryer, but they come out very well in a deep fryer.

The ketogenic diet is one such example. The diet calls for a very small number of carbs to be eaten. This means food such as rice, pasta, and other starchy vegetables like potatoes are off the menu. Even relaxed versions of the keto diet minimize carbs to a large extent and this compromises the goals of many dieters. They end up having to exert large amounts of willpower to follow the diet. This doesn't do them any favors since willpower is like a muscle. At some point, it tires and this is when the dieter goes right back to their old pattern of eating. I have personal experience with this. In terms of health benefits, the keto diet offers the most. The reduction of carbs forces your body to mobilize fat and this results in automatic fat loss and better health.

Feel free to mix and match the recipes you see in here and play around with them. Eating is supposed to be fun! Unfortunately, we've associated fun eating with unhealthy food. This doesn't have to be the case. The air fryer, combined with the Mediterranean diet, will make your mealtimes fun-filled again and full of taste. There's no grease and messy cleanups to deal with anymore. Are you excited yet?

You should be! You're about to embark on a journey full of air fried goodness!

Texas BBQ Chicken Thighs

Prep + Cook Time: 30 minutes

4 Servings

INGREDIENTS

8 chicken thighs

Salt and black pepper to taste

2 tsp Texas BBQ Jerky seasoning

1 tbsp olive oil

2 tbsp fresh cilantro, chopped

DIRECTIONS

Preheat air fryer to 380 F.

Grease the frying basket with cooking spray.

Drizzle the chicken with olive oil, season with salt and black pepper, and sprinkle with BBQ seasoning.

Place in the fryer and Bake for 15 minutes in total, flipping once.

Top with fresh cilantro to serve.

Authentic Spanish Patatas Bravas

Prep + Cook Time: 40 minutes

4 Servings

INGREDIENTS

1 lb waxy potatoes, into bite-size chunks

4 tbsp olive oil

1 tsp smoked paprika

1 shallot, chopped

2 tomatoes, chopped

1 tbsp tomato paste

1 tbsp flour

2 tbsp sriracha hot chili sauce

1 tsp sugar

2 tbsp fresh parsley, chopped

Salt to taste

DIRECTIONS

Heat 2 tbsp of the olive oil in a skillet over medium heat and sauté the shallot for 3 minutes until fragrant.

Stir in the flour for 2 more minutes.

Add in the remaining ingredients and 1 cup of water.

Bring to a boil, reduce the heat, and simmer for 6-8 minutes until the sauce becomes pulpy.

Remove to a food processor and blend until smooth.

Let cool completely.

Preheat air fryer to 400 F.

Coat potatoes with the remaining olive oil and AirFry in the fryer for 20-25 minutes, shaking once halfway through.

Sprinkle with salt and spoon over the sauce to serve.

Enjoy!

Crispy Bell Peppers with Tartare Sauce

Prep + Cook Time: 25 minutes

4 Servings

INGREDIENTS

1 egg, beaten

2 bell peppers, cut into ½-inch-thick slices

⅔ cup panko breadcrumbs

½ tsp paprika

½ tsp garlic powder

Salt to taste

1 tsp lime juice

¼ tsp Dijon mustard

½ cup mayonnaise

2 tbsp capers, chopped

2 tbsp fresh parsley

2 dill pickles, chopped

DIRECTIONS

Preheat your Air Fryer to 390 F.

Mix the panko breadcrumbs, paprika, garlic powder, and salt in a shallow bowl.

In a separate bowl, whisk the egg with 1 ½ teaspoons of water to make an egg wash.

Coat the bell pepper slices in the egg wash, then roll them in the panko mixture until fully covered.

Put the peppers in the greased air basket in a single layer and spray with olive oil, then air 4-7 minutes until light brown.

In a bowl, mix the mayonnaise, lime juice, capers, pickles, parsley, and salt.

Remove the peppers from the fryer and serve with the tartare sauce.

Enjoy!

Russian-Style Eggplant Caviar

Prep + Cook Time: 20 minutes

4 Servings

INGREDIENTS

2 eggplants

½ red onion, chopped

2 tbsp balsamic vinegar

1 tbsp olive oil

Salt to taste

DIRECTIONS

Arrange the eggplants in the greased frying basket and Bake for 15 minutes at 380 F.

Remove and let cool.

Then, cut the eggplants in half, lengthwise, and empty their insides with a spoon.

Transfer the flesh to a food processor and add in red onion and olive oil; process until smooth.

Season with balsamic vinegar and a bit of salt.

cold on a bread slice.

Enjoy!

Cheese & Cauliflower Tater Tot Bites

Prep + Cook Time: 35 minutes

4 Servings

INGREDIENTS

1large egg

¼ cup Pecorino cheese, grated

¼ cup sharp cheddar cheese, shredded

1 lb cauliflower florets

1 garlic clove, minced

½ cup seasoned breadcrumbs

1 tbsp olive oil

2 tbsp scallions, chopped

Salt and black pepper to taste

DIRECTIONS

Cook the cauliflower in boiling salted water until al dente.

Drain well and let it dry on absorbent paper for 10 minutes.

Then finely chop cauliflower and put it into a bowl.

Add in the egg, garlic, Pecorino cheese, cheddar cheese, breadcrumbs, salt, and pepper and stir to combine.

Chill for 10 minutes.

Preheat your Air Fryer to 380 F.

Shape the cauliflower mixture into bite-sized oval 'tater tots.'

Lay them in a single layer in the greased fryer basket, giving them plenty of space.

Brush the tots with oil and air fry for 15 minutes, turning halfway through the cooking time until crispy and browned.

Top with scallions and serve with your favorite sauce for dipping.

Enjoy!

Spicy Vegetable Skewers

Prep + Cook Time: 25 minutes

2 Servings

INGREDIENTS

2large sweet potatoes

1 beetroot

1 green bell pepper

1 tsp chili flakes

Salt and black pepper to taste

½ tsp turmeric

¼ tsp garlic powder

¼ tsp paprika

1 tbsp olive oil

DIRECTIONS

Preheat air fryer to 350 F.

Peel the veggies and cut them into bite-sized chunks.

Place the chunks in a bowl along with the remaining ingredients and mix until completely coated.

Thread the vegetables, alternately, onto skewers in this order: potato, pepper, and beetroot.

Place in the greased frying basket and Bake for 18-20 minutes, turning once.

Serve with yogurt dip.

Enjoy!

Classic French Ratatouille

Prep + Cook Time: 30 minutes

2 Servings

INGREDIENTS

2 tbsp olive oil

2 Roma tomatoes, thinly sliced

2 garlic cloves, minced

1 zucchini, thinly sliced

2 yellow bell peppers, sliced

1 tbsp vinegar

2 tbsp herbs de Provence

Salt and black pepper to taste

DIRECTIONS

Preheat air fryer to 390 F.

Place all ingredients in a bowl.

Season with salt and pepper and stir to coat.

Arrange them on a baking dish and place them inside the air fryer.

Bake for 15 minutes.

Serve warm. enjoy!

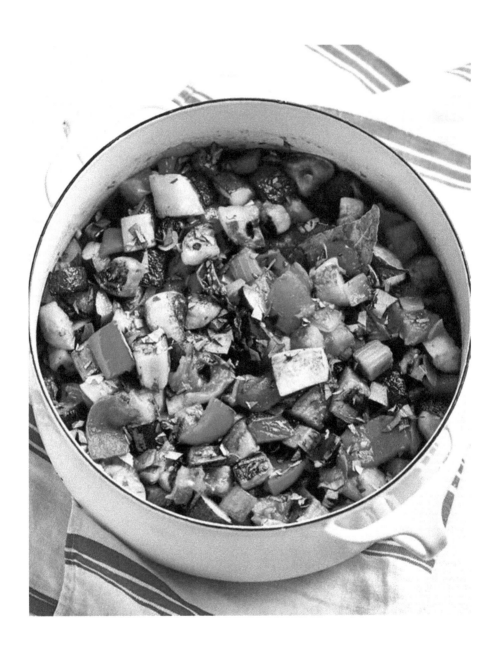

Chili Falafel with Cheesy Sauce

Prep + Cook Time: 25 minutes

4 Servings

INGREDIENTS

1 14-oz can chickpeas, drained

2 tbsp fresh parsley, chopped

6 spring onions, sliced

1 tsp garlic powder

Salt to taste

¼ tsp chili powder

1 cup cream cheese, softened

1 clove garlic, chopped

½ tsp dried dill

1 tsp hot paprika

2 tbsp olive oil

2 tbsp plain yogurt

1 tsp apple cider vinegar

DIRECTIONS

Place the cream cheese, minced garlic, dill, hot paprika, olive oil, yogurt, and vinegar in a bowl and whisk until you obtain a smooth and homogeneous sauce consistency.

Keep covered in the fridge.

In a blender, place chickpeas, parsley, spring onions, garlic powder, chili powder, and salt and process until crumbly.

Place the mixture in a bowl and refrigerate covered for 20 minutes.

For each falafel, take 2 tablespoons to form a round ball, flattened around the edges.

Preheat air fryer to 370 F and arrange falafels on the greased frying basket.

AirFry for 14-16 minutes, flipping once until lightly browned and cooked through.

Serve with the cream cheese sauce.

Enjoy!

Italian-Style Stuffed Mushrooms

Prep + Cook Time: 25 minutes

4 Servings

INGREDIENTS

4 oz mascarpone cheese, softened

1 egg

1 cup fresh baby spinach

20 large mushrooms, stems removed

¾ cup shredded Italian blend cheese

¼ cup breadcrumbs

1 tbsp olive oil

Salt and black pepper to taste

DIRECTIONS

Preheat your Air Fryer to 375 F.

Whisk the mascarpone cheese, Italian blend cheese, breadcrumbs, egg, salt, and pepper with an electric mixer.

Stir in the spinach with a spoon until everything is well combined.

Divide the mixture between the mushrooms, leaving some popping out of the top.

Put the mushrooms in the greased fryer basket and drizzle them with olive oil.

AirFry for 7-10 minutes, until the mushrooms have begun to brown and the cheese on top is light brown.

Serve warm.

Enjoy!

Air Fried Veggie Sushi

Prep + Cook Time: 30 minutes

4 Servings

INGREDIENTS

2 cups cooked sushi rice

4 nori sheets

1 carrot, sliced lengthways

1 red bell pepper, sliced

1 avocado, sliced

1 tbsp olive oil

1 tbsp rice wine vinegar

1 cup panko crumbs

2 tbsp sesame seeds

Soy sauce, wasabi, and pickled ginger to serve

DIRECTIONS

Prepare a clean working board, a small bowl of lukewarm water, and a sushi mat.

Wet your hands, and lay a nori sheet onto the sushi mat, and spread a half cup of sushi rice, leaving a half-inch of nori clear, so you can seal the roll.

Place carrot, pepper, and avocado sideways to the rice.

Roll sushi tightly and rub warm water along the clean nori strip to seal.

In a bowl, mix oil and rice vinegar.

In another bowl, mix crumbs and sesame seeds.

Roll each sushi log in the vinegar mixture and then straight to the sesame bowl to coat.

Arrange sushi in the air fryer and Bake for 14 minutes at 360 F, turning once.

Slice and serve with soy sauce, pickled ginger, and wasabi.

Enjoy!

Crispy Mozzarella Rolls

Prep + Cook Time: 20 minutes

4 Servings

INGREDIENTS

1 lb mozzarella cheese, chopped

3 packages Pepperidge farm rolls

1 tbsp butter, softened

1 tsp mustard seeds

1 tsp poppy seeds

1 small onion, chopped

DIRECTIONS

In a bowl, mix butter, mustard seeds, onion, and poppy seeds.

Spread the mixture on top of the rolls.

Cover with cheese, roll up, and arrange on the greased frying basket.

Bake at 350 F for 15 minutes.

Enjoy!

Brussels Sprouts with Raisins & Pine Nuts

Prep + Cook Time: 20 minutes

4 Servings

INGREDIENTS

1 lb Brussels sprouts, stems cut off and halved

2 tbsp olive oil

1 ¾ oz raisins, soaked and drained

Juice of 1 orange

Salt to taste

2 tbsp pine nuts, toasted

DIRECTIONS

Preheat air fryer to 390 F.

In a bowl, toss the Brussels sprouts with olive oil and salt and stir to combine.

Place in the frying and Bake for 15 minutes, shaking once halfway through.

Top with toasted pine nuts and raisins.

Drizzle with orange juice to serve.

Serve.

Enjoy!

Spicy Sweet Potato French Fries

Prep + Cook Time: 30 minutes

4 Servings

INGREDIENTS

½ tsp salt

½ tsp garlic powder

½ tsp chili powder

¼ tsp cumin

3 tbsp olive oil

4 sweet potatoes, cut into thick strips

DIRECTIONS

In a bowl, mix salt, garlic powder, chili powder, and cumin and whisk in olive oil.

Coat the strips in the mixture and place them in the frying basket.

AirFry for 20 minutes at 380 F, shaking once, until crispy.

Traditional Jacket Potatoes

Prep + Cook Time: 30 minutes

4 Servings

INGREDIENTS

1 lb potatoes

2 garlic cloves, minced

Salt and black pepper to taste

1 tsp dried rosemary

2 tsp butter, melted

DIRECTIONS

Preheat air fryer to 360 F.

Prick the potatoes with a fork.

Place them in the greased frying basket and Bake for 23-25 minutes, turning once halfway through.

Remove and cut in half.

Drizzle with melted butter and season with salt and black pepper.

Sprinkle with rosemary and serve.

Enjoy!

Green Cabbage with Blue Cheese Sauce

Prep + Cook Time: 25 minutes

4 Servings

INGREDIENTS

1 head green cabbage, cut into wedges

1 cup mozzarella cheese, shredded

4 tbsp butter, melted

Salt and black pepper to taste

½ cup blue cheese sauce

DIRECTIONS

Preheat air fryer to 380 F.

Brush cabbage wedges with butter and sprinkle with mozzarella.

Transfer to a greased baking dish and Bake in the air fryer for 20 minutes.

Serve with blue cheese sauce.

Enjoy!

Eggplant & Zucchini Chips

Prep + Cook Time: 20 minutes

4 Servings

INGREDIENTS

1 large eggplant, cut into strips

1 zucchini, cut into strips

½ cup cornstarch

3 tbsp olive oil

Salt to season

DIRECTIONS

Preheat air fryer to 390 F.

In a bowl, stir in cornstarch, salt, pepper, olive oil, eggplants, and zucchini.

Place the coated veggies in the greased frying basket and AirFry for 12 minutes, shaking once.

Enjoy!

Cholula Seasoned Broccoli

Prep + Cook Time: 30 minutes

4 Servings

INGREDIENTS

1 lb broccoli florets

½ tsp lemon zest

1 garlic clove, minced

1 tsp olive oil

1 ½ tbsp soy sauce

1 tsp lemon juice

1 tsp cholula hot sauce

Salt and black pepper to taste

DIRECTIONS

Preheat your Air Fryer to 390 F.

Put the broccoli florets, olive oil, and garlic in a bowl and season with salt.

Toss together, then put the broccoli in the greased fryer basket, giving the florets plenty of space.

Air fry for 15-20 minutes or until light brown and crispy.

Shake the basket every 5 minutes.

Whisk the soy sauce, white vinegar, cholula sauce, and lemon juice in a bowl.

Toss the broccoli and sauce mixture in a large bowl and mix well.

Sprinkle with lemon zest, salt, and pepper, and serve.

Enjoy!

Spicy Mixed Veggie Bake

Prep + Cook Time: 35 minutes

4 Servings

INGREDIENTS

1 cauliflower, cut into florets

1 carrot, diced

1 broccoli, cut into florets

1 onion, chopped

½ cup garden peas

1 leek, sliced thinly

1 small zucchini, chopped

1 tbsp garlic paste

2 tbsp olive oil

1 tbsp curry paste

1 tsp dried coriander

1 tsp ground cumin

1 cup vegetable broth

1 tsp ginger paste

Salt and black pepper to taste

DIRECTIONS

Preheat air fryer to 350 F.

Heat olive oil in a saucepan over medium heat and sauté onion, leek, ginger paste, carrot, curry paste, and garlic for 5 minutes.

Stir in the remaining ingredients and transfer to a baking dish.

Bake in the air fryer for 10-15 minutes. Serve warm. enjoy!

Air Fried Ravioli

Prep + Cook Time: 15 minutes

4 Servings

INGREDIENTS

1 package cheese ravioli

2 cup Italian breadcrumbs

¼ cup Pecorino cheese, grated

1 cup buttermilk

2 tsp olive oil

¼ tsp garlic powder

DIRECTIONS

Preheat air fryer to 390 F.

In a small bowl, combine breadcrumbs, Pecorino cheese, garlic powder, and olive oil.

Dip the ravioli in the buttermilk and then coat them with the breadcrumb mixture.

Line a baking tray with parchment paper and arrange the ravioli on it.

Place in the air fryer and Bake for 5-6 minutes.

Serve with marinara or carbonara sauce.

enjoy!

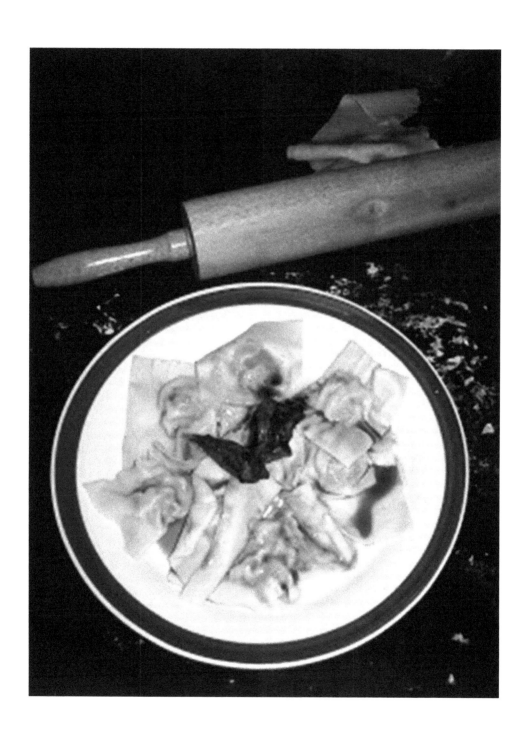

43

Hoisin Spring Rolls

Prep + Cook Time: 25 minutes

4 Servings

INGREDIENTS

½ lb shiitake mushrooms, chopped

2 tbsp canola oil

1 clove garlic, minced

1-inch piece ginger, grated

2 cups green cabbage, shredded

1 carrot, shredded

1 green onion, thinly sliced

1 tbsp soy sauce

1 tbsp hoisin sauce

12 wonton wrappers

DIRECTIONS

Warm 1 tbsp of the canola oil in a pan over medium heat and sauté green onion, garlic, and ginger for 30 seconds.

Add in shiitake mushrooms, carrots, and cabbage and cook, stirring occasionally until tender, about 4 minutes.

Stir in the soy sauce and hoisin sauce.

Preheat air fryer to 390 F.

Distribute the mixture across the wrappers and roll-up.

Place the rolls in the greased frying basket and Bake for 14-16 minutes, turning once until golden and crisp.

Serve warm.

Enjoy!

Greek-Style Stuffed Bell Peppers

Prep + Cook Time: 20 minutes

4 Servings

INGREDIENTS

4 red bell peppers, tops sliced off

2 cups cooked rice

1 onion, chopped

1 tbsp Greek seasoning

¼ cup Kalamata olives, pitted and sliced

¾ cup tomato sauce

Salt and black pepper to taste

1 cup feta cheese, crumbled

2 tbsp fresh dill, chopped

DIRECTIONS

Preheat air fryer to 360 F.

Microwave the bell peppers for 1-2 minutes until soft.

In a bowl, combine rice, onion, Greek seasoning, feta cheese, olives, tomato sauce, salt, and pepper.

Divide the mixture between the bell peppers and arrange them on a greased baking dish.

Place in the air fryer and Bake for 15 minutes.

When ready, remove to a serving plate, scatter with dill and serve.

Enjoy!

Cheesy Vegetable Quesadilla

Prep + Cook Time: 15 minutes

1 Servings

INGREDIENTS

2 flour tortillas

¼ cup gouda cheese, shredded

¼ yellow bell pepper, sliced

¼ zucchini, sliced

½ green onion, sliced

1 tbsp fresh cilantro, chopped

1 tsp olive oil

DIRECTIONS

Preheat air fryer to 390 F.

Grease the air fryer basket with cooking spray.

Place a flour tortilla in the greased frying basket and top with gouda cheese, bell pepper, zucchini, cilantro, and green onion.

Cover with the other tortilla and brush with olive oil.

Cook for 10 minutes until lightly browned.

Cut into 4 wedges and serve.

enjoy!

Cheesy Broccoli & Egg Cups

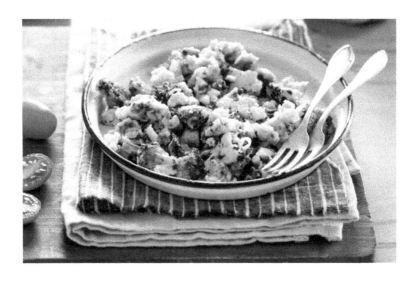

Prep + Cook Time: 15 minutes

4 Servings

INGREDIENTS

1 lb broccoli florets, steamed and chopped

4 eggs, beaten

1 cup sharp cheese, shredded

1 cup heavy cream

½ tsp nutmeg

½ tsp ginger powder

Salt and black pepper to taste

DIRECTIONS

Place the broccoli in a bowl and mix in eggs, heavy cream, nutmeg, ginger, salt, and black pepper.

Divide the mixture between 4 greased ramekins.

Top with the cheese and Bake in the air fryer for 12-14 minutes at 330 F.

Remove and let cool for a few minutes before serving. enjoy!

Potato Filled Bread Rolls

Prep + Cook Time: 25 minutes

4 Servings

INGREDIENTS

8 slices sandwich bread

4 large potatoes, boiled and mashed

½ tsp turmeric

2 green chilies, seeded and chopped

1 onion, finely chopped

½ tsp mustard seeds

1 tbsp olive oil Salt to taste

DIRECTIONS

Preheat air fryer to 350 F.

In a skillet over medium heat, warm olive oil, and stir-fry onion and mustard seeds for 3 minutes.

Remove to a bowl and add in potatoes, chilies, turmeric, and salt; mix well.

Trim the crust sides of the bread, and roll out with a rolling pin.

Spread a spoonful of the potato mixture on each bread sheet, and roll the bread over the filling, sealing the edges.

Place the rolls in the greased frying basket and Bake for 12 minutes.

Serve warm.

enjoy!

Roasted Brussels Sprouts

Prep + Cook Time: 25 minutes

4 Servings

INGREDIENTS

1 lb Brussels sprouts

1 tsp garlic powder

2 tbsp olive oil

Salt and black pepper to taste

DIRECTIONS

Trim off the outer leaves, keeping only the head of the Brussels sprouts.

In a bowl, mix olive oil, garlic powder, salt, and pepper.

Add in the sprouts and coat well.

Transfer them to the greased frying basket and AirFry for 15 minutes, shaking once halfway through.

Serve warm.

Enjoy!

Sesame Balsamic Asparagus

Prep + Cook Time: 25 minutes

4 Servings

INGREDIENTS

1 ½ lb asparagus, trimmed

4 tbsp balsamic vinegar

4 tbsp olive oil

2 tbsp fresh rosemary, chopped

Salt and black pepper to taste

2 tbsp sesame seeds

DIRECTIONS

Preheat your Air Fryer to 360 F.

Whisk the olive oil, sesame seeds, and balsamic vinegar to make a marinade in a bowl.

Place the asparagus on a baking dish and pour over the asparagus the marinade.

Toss to coat and let them sit for 10 minutes.

Then AirFry for 10-12 minutes, shaking halfway through the cooking time until tender and lighty charred.

Serve asparagus topped with rosemary.

Enjoy!

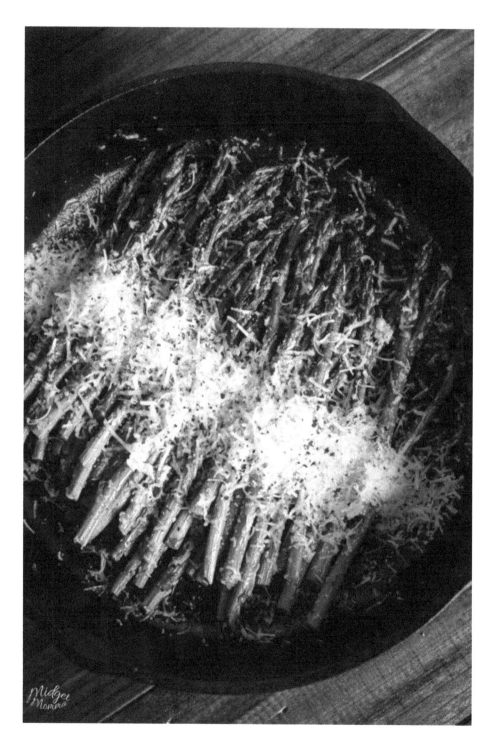

57

Easy Roasted Cauliflower

Prep + Cook Time: 30 minutes

4 Servings

INGREDIENTS

1 head cauliflower, cut into florets

1 tsp garlic powder

1 tsp turmeric

1 tsp cumin

1 tbsp olive oil

Salt and black pepper to taste

DIRECTIONS

Preheat your Air Fryer to 390 F.

Thoroughly combine the cauliflower florets, turmeric, cumin, and garlic powder in a mixing bowl; toss to coat the florets well.

Add salt and pepper to taste.

Add the cauliflower to the greased fryer basket and brush with olive oil.

Air fry until browned and crispy, about 20 minutes.

Be sure to shake the basket every 5 minutes or so.

Serve hot.

enjoy!

Winter Vegetable Delight

Prep + Cook Time: 20 minutes

2 Servings

INGREDIENTS

1 parsnip, sliced

1 cup sliced butternut squash

1 small red onion, cut into wedges

½ celery stalk, chopped

1 tbsp fresh thyme, chopped

Salt and black pepper to taste

2 tsp olive oil

DIRECTIONS

Preheat air fryer to 380 F.

In a bowl, add turnip, squash, onion, celery, thyme, pepper, salt, and olive oil; mix well.

Pour the vegetables into the frying basket and AirFry for 16 minutes, tossing once.

Serve.

enjoy!

Roasted Veggies with Penne Pasta

Prep + Cook Time: 45 minutes

4 Servings

INGREDIENTS

1lb penne pasta 1 zucchini, sliced

1 bell pepper, sliced

½ lb acorn squash, sliced

½ cup mushrooms, sliced

½ cup Kalamata olives, pitted and halved

¼ cup olive oil

1 tsp Italian seasoning

1 cup grape tomatoes, halved

3 tbsp balsamic vinegar

2 tbsp fresh basil, chopped

Salt and black pepper to taste

DIRECTIONS

Fill a pot with salted water and bring to a boil over medium heat.

Add in the penne pasta and cook until al dente, about 8 minutes.

Drain and place in a bowl; set aside.

Preheat air fryer to 380 F.

In a baking dish, combine bell pepper, zucchini, acorn squash, mushrooms, and olive oil.

Season with salt and pepper.

Bake in the air fryer for 15 minutes, shaking once.

Remove the veggies to the pasta bowl.

Mix in tomatoes, olives, Italian seasoning, and balsamic vinegar.

Sprinkle with basil and serve.

enjoy!

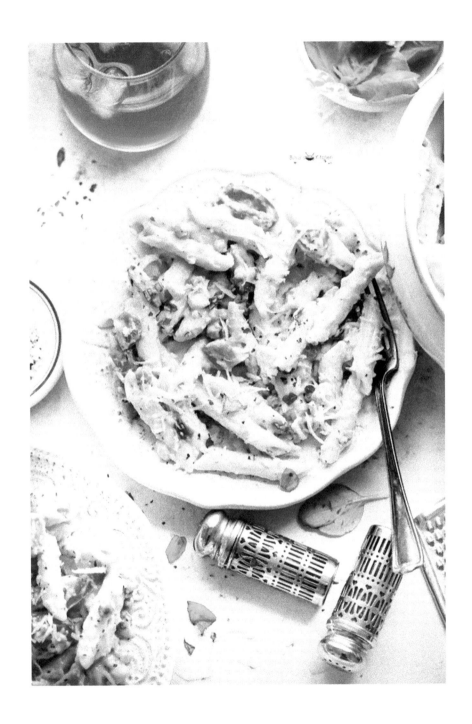

Mexican Chile Relleno

Prep + Cook Time: 20 minutes

4 Servings

INGREDIENTS

2 8-oz cans whole green chiles,drained

2 cups Mexican cheese, shredded

1 cup flour

2 large eggs, beaten

½ cup milk

DIRECTIONS

Preheat air fryer to 380 F.

Lay the green chilies on a plate and fill them with cheese.

In a bowl, whisk eggs, milk, and half of the flour.

Pour the remaining flour on a flat plate.

Dip the chilies in the flour first, then in the egg mixture, and arrange them on the greased frying basket.

AirFry for 8-10 minutes, flipping once halfway through.

Serve with slices of avocado.

Enjoy!

Plantain Fritters

Prep + Cook Time: 15 minutes

4 Servings

INGREDIENTS

3 bananas, sliced diagonally

2 tbsp cornflour

1 egg white

¼ cup breadcrumbs

Salt and black pepper to taste

DIRECTIONS

Preheat air fryer to 340 F.

Pour breadcrumbs on a plate.

Season with salt and pepper.

Coat the plantain slices with the cornflour first, brush with egg white, and roll in the breadcrumbs.

Arrange on a greased baking tray and lightly spray with oil.

Bake in the air fryer for 8 minutes, flipping once. Serve. enjoy!

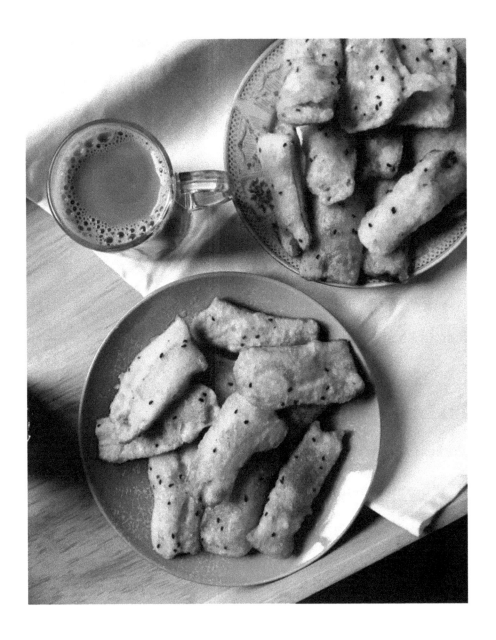

Spanish-Style Huevos Rotos Broken Eggs

Prep + Cook Time: 36 minutes

2 Servings

INGREDIENTS

½ tsp salt

½ tsp garlic powder

3 tbsp olive oil

1 tsp sweet paprika

2 russet potatoes, cut into wedges

2 eggs

DIRECTIONS

In a bowl, mix salt, garlic powder, and 1 tbsp olive oil.

Add in the potatoes and toss to coat.

Arrange them on the frying basket without overcrowding and AirFry for 20-25 minutes at 380 F.

Shake regularly to get crispy on all sides.

Heat the remaining olive oil in a pan over medium heat and fry the eggs until the whites are firm and the yolks are still runny, about 5 minutes.

Place the potatoes on a serving bowl and top with the fried eggs and paprika.

Break the eggs with a fork and serve.

enjoy!

Traditional Jacket Potatoes

Prep + Cook Time: 30 minutes

4 Servings

INGREDIENTS

1 lb potatoes

2 garlic cloves, minced

Salt and black pepper to taste

1 tsp dried rosemary

2 tsp butter, melted

DIRECTIONS

Preheat air fryer to 360 F.

Prick the potatoes with a fork.

Place them in the greased frying basket and Bake for 23-25 minutes, turning once halfway through.

Remove and cut in half.

Drizzle with melted butter and season with salt and black pepper. Sprinkle with rosemary and serve enjoy!.

Easy Cabbage Steaks

Prep + Cook Time:25 minutes

3 Servings

INGREDIENTS

1 cabbage head

1 tbsp garlic paste

2 tbsp olive oil

Salt and black pepper to taste

2 tsp fennel seeds

DIRECTIONS

Preheat air fryer to 350 F.

Cut the cabbage into 1 ½-inch thin slices.

In a small bowl, combine all the other ingredients and brush cabbage with the mixture.

Arrange the steaks on the greased frying basket and Bake for 15 minutes, flipping once halfway through.

Serve warm or chilled. enjoy!

Zesty Bell Pepper Bites

Prep + Cook Time: 20 minutes

4 Servings

INGREDIENTS

1 red bell pepper, cut into small portions

1 yellow pepper, cut into small portions

1 green bell pepper, cut into small portions

3 tbsp balsamic vinegar

2 tbsp olive oil

1 garlic clove, minced

½ tsp dried basil

½ tsp dried parsley Salt and black pepper to taste

½ cup garlic mayonnaise

DIRECTIONS

Preheat air fryer to 390 F.

In a bowl, mix bell peppers, olive oil, garlic, balsamic vinegar, basil, and parsley and season with salt and black pepper.

Transfer to a greased baking dish and Bake in the air fryer for 12-15 minutes, tossing once or twice.

Serve with garlic mayonnaise.

enjoy!

Indian Fried Okra

Prep + Cook Time:20 minutes

4 Servings

INGREDIENTS

1 tbsp chili powder

2 tbsp garam masala

1 cup cornmeal

¼ cup flour Salt to taste

½ lb okra, trimmed and halved lengthwise

1 egg

DIRECTIONS

Preheat air fryer to 380 F.

In a bowl, mix cornmeal, flour, chili powder, garam masala, salt, and pepper.

In another bowl, whisk the egg; season with salt and pepper.

Dip the okra in the egg and then coat in cornmeal mixture.

Spray okra with cooking spray and place in the frying basket.

AirFry for 6 minutes, slide the basket out, shake and cook for another 6 minutes until golden brown.

 Serve with hot sauce.

enjoy!

Cheesy Eggplant Schnitzels

Prep + Cook Time:15 minutes

4 Servings

INGREDIENTS

2eggplants

½ cup mozzarella cheese, grated

2 tbsp milk

1 egg, beaten

2 cups breadcrumbs

2 tomatoes, sliced

DIRECTIONS

Preheat air fryer to 400 F.

Cut the eggplants lengthways into ½-in thick slices.

In a bowl, mix egg and milk.

In another bowl, combine breadcrumbs and mozzarella cheese.

Dip eggplant slices in the egg mixture, followed by the crumb mixture.

Place in the greased frying basket and AirFry for 10-12 minutes, turning once halfway through.

Top with tomato slices and serve.

enjoy!

Air Fried Eggplant Toast

Prep + Cook Time: 12 minutes

2 Servings

INGREDIENTS

2 large eggplant slices

1 large spring onion, finely sliced

2 white bread slices

½ cup sweet corn

1 egg white, whisked

1 tbsp black sesame seeds

DIRECTIONS

In a bowl, place corn, spring onion, egg white, and sesame seeds and mix well.

Spread the mixture over the bread slices.

Top with eggplants and place in the greased air fryer basket.

Bake for 8-10 minutes at 370 F until golden.

Serve enjoy!

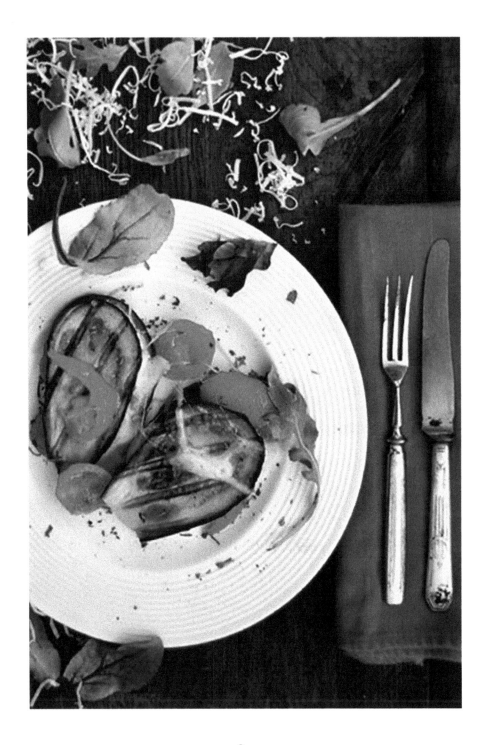

Tasty Balsamic Beets

Prep + Cook Time: 25 minutes

2 Servings

INGREDIENTS

2 beets, cubed

⅓ cup balsamic vinegar

2 tbsp olive oil

1 tbsp honey

Salt and black pepper to taste

2 springs rosemary, chopped

DIRECTIONS

Preheat air fryer to 400 F.

In a bowl, mix beets, olive oil, rosemary, pepper, and salt and toss to coat.

Bake the beets in the frying basket for 15 minutes, shaking once halfway through.

Pour the balsamic vinegar and honey into a pan over medium heat; bring to a boil and cook until reduced by half.

Drizzle the beets with balsamic sauce and serve.

enjoy!

Teriyaki Cauliflower

Prep + Cook Time:20 minutes

4 Servings

INGREDIENTS

1 big cauliflower head, cut into florets

½ cup soy sauce

1 tbsp brown sugar

1 tsp sesame oil

½ chili powder

2 cloves garlic, chopped

1 tsp cornstarch

DIRECTIONS

In a bowl, whisk soy sauce, sugar, sesame oil, ⅓ cup of water, chili powder, garlic, and cornstarch until smooth.

In a bowl, add cauliflower and pour teriyaki sauce over the top, toss to coat.

Place the cauliflower in the greased frying basket and AirFry for 14 minutes at 340 F, turning once halfway through.

When ready, check if the cauliflower is cooked but not too soft.

Serve warm.

enjoy!

Chili Corn on the Cob

Prep + Cook Time: 25 minutes

4 Servings

INGREDIENTS

4 ears of sweet corn, shucked

1 clove garlic, minced

1 green chili, minced

1 lemon, zested

2 tbsp olive oil

2 tbsp butter, melted

Salt to taste

DIRECTIONS

Preheat air fryer to 380 F.

in a bowl, mix olive oil, garlic, lemon zest, and green chili.

Rub the mixture on all sides.

Place the ears in the frying basket; work in batches.

AirFry for 14-16 minutes, turning once until lightly browned.

Remove to a platter and drizzle with melted butter.

Scatter with salt and serve.

enjoy!

Vegetable Bean Burgers

Prep + Cook Time: 45 minutes

4 Servings

INGREDIENTS

1 parsnip, chopped

1 carrot, chopped

½ lb mushrooms, chopped

1 15-oz can black beans, drained and rinsed

2 tbsp olive oil

1 egg, beaten

2 tbsp tomato paste

2 garlic cloves, minced

½ tsp onion powder ½ cup breadcrumbs

Salt and black pepper to taste

4 hamburger buns

DIRECTIONS

Preheat your Air Fryer to 360 F.

Put the parsnip and carrot in the greased fryer basket, drizzle with some olive oil, and season with salt and pepper.

AirFry for 8 minutes.

Toss the mushrooms in the fryer basket with the veggies, spray with oil, and season with salt and pepper.

AirFry for 5 more minutes.

Mash the black beans in a bowl with a fork.

Mix in the egg, tomato paste, garlic, onion powder, salt, cooked carrots, and mushrooms and mash the veggies with a fork.

Add the breadcrumbs and stir to combine.

Make 4 patties out of the mixture.

Put the patties in the fryer basket, giving each patty plenty of room.

AirFry for 5 minutes, flip and spray with oil, then air fry for 5-7 more minutes.

Serve on buns.

enjoy!

Nutty Pumpkin with Blue Cheese

Prep + Cook Time: 30 minutes

2 Servings

INGREDIENTS

½ small pumpkin, chopped

2 oz blue cheese, crumbled

2 tbsp pine nuts, toasted

1 tbsp olive oil

½ cup baby spinach, packed

1 spring onion, sliced

2 radishes, thinly sliced

1 tsp white wine vinegar

DIRECTIONS

Preheat air fryer to 390 F.

Place the pumpkin on a baking dish and drizzle with the olive oil; toss well.

Bake in the air fryer for 20 minutes, shaking once.

Remove to a serving bowl. Add in baby spinach, radishes, and spring onion; drizzle with vinegar.

Top with blue cheese and pine nuts to serve warm. enjoy!

Garlicky Vegetable Spread

Prep + Cook Time: 20 minutes

6 Servings

INGREDIENTS

1 lb green peppers

1 lb tomatoes

1 medium onion

3 tbsp olive oil

½ tbsp salt

4 galic cloves, peeled

DIRECTIONS

Preheat air fryer to 360 F.

Place green peppers, tomatoes, and onion in the greased frying basket and Bake for 5 minutes, flip, and cook for 10 more minutes.

Remove and peel the skin.

Place the vegetables in a blender and add the garlic, olive oil, and salt and pulse until smooth.

Serve. enjoy!

Crispy Fried Tofu

Prep + Cook Time: 20 minutes

4 Servings

INGREDIENTS

14 oz firm tofu, cut into ½-inch thick strips

2 tbsp olive oil

½ cup flour

½ cup crushed cornflakes

 Salt and black pepper to taste

DIRECTIONS

On a plate, mix flour, cornflakes, salt, and black pepper.

Dip each tofu strip into the mixture to coat, brush with oil, and arrange them on the frying basket.

Bake for 14 minutes at 360 F, turning once.

enjoy!

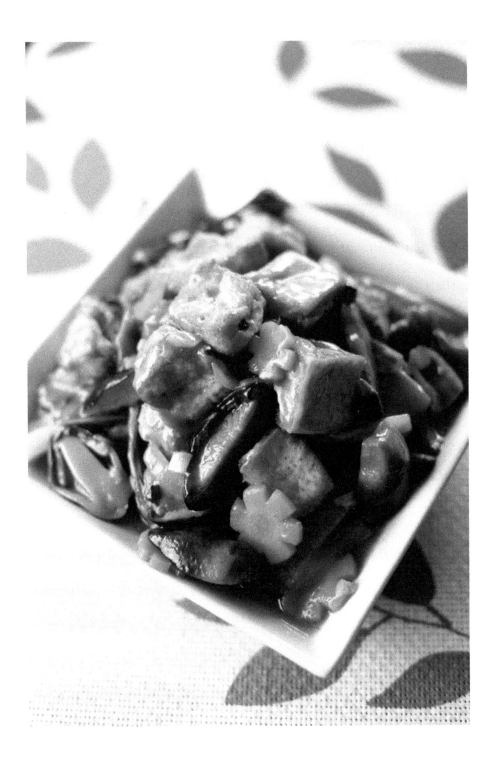

Fava Bean Falafel with Tzatziki

Prep + Cook Time: 25 minutes

4 Servings

INGREDIENTS

2 cups cooked fava beans

½ cup flour

2 tbsp fresh parsley, chopped

Juice of 1 lemon

2 garlic cloves, chopped

1 onion, chopped

½ tsp ground cumin

1 cup tzatziki sauce

4 pita wraps, warm

Salt and black pepper to taste

DIRECTIONS

In a blender, add chickpeas, flour, parsley, lemon juice, garlic, onion, cumin, salt, and pepper and blend until well-combined but not too battery; there should be some lumps.

Shape the mixture into balls.

Press them with hands, making sure they are still around.

Spray with olive oil and arrange on a paper-lined air fryer basket.

AirFry for 14 minutes at 360 F, turning once halfway through until crunchy and golden.

Serve in the pita wraps drizzled with tzatziki sauce. enjoy!

Eggplant Gratin with Mozzarella Crust

Prep + Cook Time: 30 minutes

2 Servings

INGREDIENTS

1 cup eggplants, cubed

¼ cup red peppers, chopped

¼ cup green peppers, chopped

¼ cup onion, chopped

⅓ cup tomatoes, chopped

1 garlic clove, minced

1 tbsp sliced pimiento-stuffed olives

1 tsp capers

¼ tsp dried basil

¼ tsp dried marjoram Salt and black pepper to taste

¼ cup mozzarella cheese, grated

1 tbsp breadcrumbs

DIRECTIONS

Preheat air fryer to 300 F.

In a bowl, add eggplants, green peppers, red peppers, onion, tomatoes, olives, garlic, basil, marjoram, capers, salt, and pepper; mix well.

Spoon the eggplant mixture into a greased baking dish and level it using the vessel.

Sprinkle mozzarella cheese on top and cover with breadcrumbs.

Place the dish in the air fryer and Bake for 15-20 minutes. Serve warm.

enjoy!

Poblano & Tomato Stuffed Squash

Prep + Cook Time: 30 minutes

4 Servings

INGREDIENTS

1 butternut squash

6 grape tomatoes, halved

1 poblano pepper, cut into strips

¼ cup mozzarella cheese, grated

2 tsp olive oil

Salt and black pepper to taste

DIRECTIONS

Preheat air fryer to 350 F.

Trim the ends and cut the squash lengthwise.

You will only need one half for this recipe.

Scoop the flesh out to make room for the filling.

Brush the squash with olive oil.

Place in the air fryer and Bake for 15 minutes.

Combine the remaining olive oil with tomatoes and poblano pepper, season with salt and pepper.

Fill the squash half with the mixture and Bake for 12 more minutes.

Top with mozzarella cheese and cook further for 3 minutes until the cheese melts.

enjoy!

Jalapeño & Bean Tacos

Prep + Cook Time: 25 minutes

4 Servings

INGREDIENTS

4 soft taco shells, warm

½ cup kidney beans, drained

½ cup black beans, drained

1 tbsp tomato puree

1 fresh jalapeño pepper, chopped

2 tbsp fresh cilantro, chopped

1 cup corn kernels

½ tsp cumin

½ tsp cayenne pepper

Salt and black pepper to taste

1 cup mozzarella cheese, grated

Guacamole to serve

DIRECTIONS

In a bowl, add kidney and black beans, tomato puree, jalapeño, cilantro, corn, cumin, cayenne, salt, and pepper and stir.

Fill taco shells with the bean mixture and sprinkle with mozzarella.

Lay the tacos on the greased frying basket and Bake for 14 minutes at 360 F, turning once.

Serve with guacamole.

enjoy!

Sweet & Tangy Chicken

Preparation Time: 10 minutes

Cooking Time: 15 minutes

Serve: 3

Ingredients:

1 lb chicken breast, boneless and cut into bite-size pieces

1 tbsp sesame seeds, toasted

2 garlic cloves, minced

1tsp fresh ginger, chopped

1 tsp orange zest, grated

2 tbsp orange juice

1 tbsp sesame oil

2 tbsp vinegar

1/4 cup coconut amino

1 tsp garlic powder

3 1/2 tbsp arrowroot

Directions:

Toss chicken with 3 tablespoons of arrowroot and garlic powder.

Place the cooking tray in the air fryer basket.

Select Air Fry mode.

Set time to 12 minutes and temperature 370 F then press START.

The air fryer display will prompt you to ADD FOOD once the temperature is reached then add chicken pieces in the air fryer basket.

Spray chicken pieces with cooking spray.

Toss chicken halfway through.

Meanwhile, for sauce, in a small saucepan, whisk together vinegar, garlic, ginger, orange zest, sesame oil, orange juice, and coconut aminos.

Whisk in remaining arrowroot and cook over medium heat until sauce thicken.

Remove from heat.

Once the chicken is done, toss in a mixing bowl with sauce.

Sprinkle with sesame seeds and serve.

Garlic Herb Turkey Breast

Preparation Time: 10 minutes

Cooking Time: 40 minutes

Serve: 6

Ingredients:

3 lbs turkey breast, boneless & thawed

2 garlic cloves, minced

1 tbsp fresh parsley, chopped

1 tbsp fresh rosemary, chopped

1 tsp pepper 1 tsp salt

Directions:

In a small bowl, mix together garlic, parsley, rosemary, pepper, and salt and rub all over turkey breast.

Place the cooking tray in the air fryer basket.

Select Air Fry mode.

Set time to 40 minutes and temperature 350 F then press START.

The air fryer display will prompt you to ADD FOOD once the temperature is reached then place turkey breast in the air fryer basket.

Remove turkey breast from the air fryer and let it cool for 10 minutes.

Slice and serve.

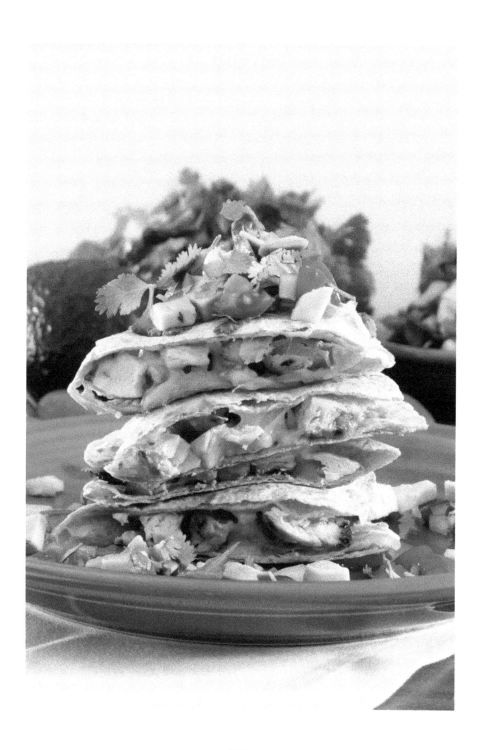

.